ANGER

A Simple & Practical Approach for Those Who Need a Better Way of Dealing with It!

by

Carol L Rickard, LCSW, TTS

As Featured:

DR.OZ
THE GOOD LIFE

Louisiana *radio*
network

THE DR.
OZ
SHOW

esperanza
hope to cope with anxiety and depression

Doctor Health
Hawaii's #1 Health Talk Show • est. 1990

ISBN: 978-1-947745-00-1

ANGER:

A Simple & Practical Approach for Those Who Need A Better Way of Dealing With It!

by Carol L Rickard, LCSW, TTS

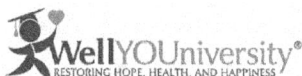

WellYOUniversity®
RESTORING HOPE, HEALTH, AND HAPPINESS

888 LIFE TOOLS (543-3866)

Carol@WellYOUniversity.com

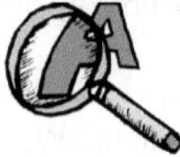

What will you get out of this book?

- A new way of *looking at* & *seeing* anger!

- Increased awareness of WHAT *anger is.*

- Simple tools for dealing with it a better way!

- Improved **quality of life**:
  your health, your relationship, your work!

Contents

Welcome

If you are reading this book,

it means *either*

YOU or someone close to you

is in need of a ***better way*** of dealing with:

Anger

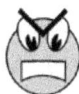

I am glad you picked up this book!

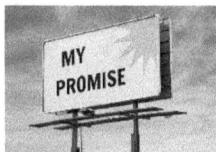

My promise to you *is this:*

By the time you get done reading,

You'll be **better prepared** to deal with

the most powerful emotion we have:

ANGER!

What this 📖 won't do:

It **WILL NOT** be 'a magic wand'.

It **WILL NOT** get any person to 'change'.

It **WILL NOT** give you 'a quick fix'.

It **WILL NOT** *even* give you 'a fix'.

What this 📖 WILL do:

Give you the **tools**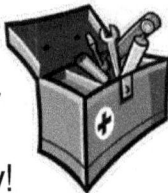
to begin managing anger
in a positive & healthy way!

About This Book

I doubt you have ever read a like this!

Unless, of course, you may have read

any of my **9** other books.

Along with **simple** & easy to understand

chapters, I tend to use a lot of pictures,

analogies, & word art

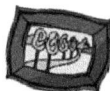

to make the information stick in the brain!

I call my approach:

SMARTheory™

It's what makes my books and services

different from all others!

KNOWLEDGE is the left brain at work.

This is where YOU *know* what to do!

Because I use "pictures" & "images", I end up

tapping in to the other side of the brain –

the right side!

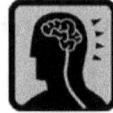

This is also the side that synthesizes things,

like the operating system in a computer!

With both sides working on the 'same page',

the end result is getting people to

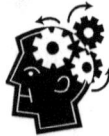

Move knowledge in to ACTION!

So, not only will you *learn*

how to manage anger in a better way,

you'll *USE* what you learn!

If you're not 100% satisfied when you finish reading,

let me know & I will refund your purchase price!

This book is divided in to *three parts:*

Part 1 will introduce you to some of my

Key Foundations

Here we'll focus on **HOW** to get started

& how to ensure your success

from the very beginning!

You'll also learn the important
difference between

Feelings & Behaviors

Part 2 we'll focus on **WHAT**

The goal being for you to get to KNOW *your* anger!

The 3 key areas you'll discover:

Vocabulary

Style

Pattern

Part 3 we'll focus on **HOW** to manage it

We'll take what you learned in Part 2 & use it to

build out your Anger Mastery Tool Box!

I will introduce you to the "tools" I've used & been

teaching to others for the past **25** years...

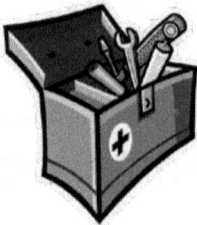

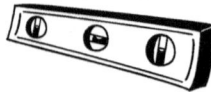

By the time we've made it thru all 3 parts -

You'll not only be able to **SEE**

your anger for the 1st time,

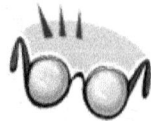

You'll also have some *practical tools* you can use to

"Deal with anger in a better way!"

WHY I Wrote This Book!

For over **25** years I've been helping people change their behaviors, habits, and health.

The problem was:

A person had to end up at a *crisis point,*

either **hospitalized** or *one step away from it…*

I've always told my patients they were the

lucky ones

because they got to learn through our program

the tools **EVERYONE** *needs to learn!*

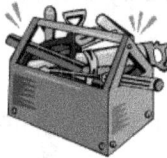

So for me, writing books, or as I like to think of them

"workshops to go"

is one way I can get these tools to people

BEFORE they *end up in a crisis.*

This particular book is based on a live workshop

I've done over the years called:

How to Be Angry **WITHOUT**:

Getting Fired

Ruining Relationships

Getting Sick!

After all, these are the 3 main areas in one's life

greatly impacted by **unmanaged anger**:

WORK

RELATIONSHIPS

HEALTH

Why Listen to Me?

I know what it's like to struggle with anger.

At 14, I started stealing alcohol from my parents.

I found out my dad was dying from cancer –

(Which I wasn't supposed to know & I didn't tell I did.)

I remember being **ANGRY** at:

EVERYONE & EVERYTHING…

Drinking:

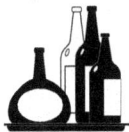

was a way I dealt the ANGER.

Luckily,

The drinking only lasted for about 6 months……

Then basketball became my way to deal!

It served me well!

I went college on a basketball scholarship.

I often say that **basketball SAVED MY LIFE.**

But after I stopped playing basketball,

I found another unhealthy way of dealing with anger:

HOLDING IT IN

And that's when my migraines became a

constant presence in my life.

As you will see, there are a couple different ways

people deal with anger in

Unhealthy Ways

It's not just those who EXPLODE!

Thank goodness I started

seeing a new doctor!

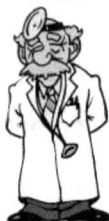

He helped me realize that I *WASN'T* managing my

anger very well in **SOME areas of my life...**

I loved my job & working with the patients.....

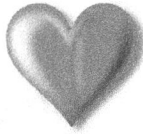

BUT my coworkers were a
constant source of anger...

I realized my *old way* of dealing with them

WAS NOT WORKING...

and I *needed to make some changes!*

So, I made a focused effort to start using

the tools & **strategies** I'd been teaching!

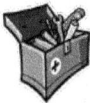

These are the same tools & strategies
I share with you here today!

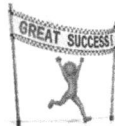

And just as they have guided me to great success –

I know they can do the same for you!

A Quick Check-In!

Just as I do in my live events, I want to have you

measure

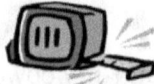

to see where you are starting from!

Circle the number below each statement that best

describes where you are RIGHT NOW!

1) I feel I have enough healthy anger tools.

0	1	2	3	4	5
not at all!					absolutely

2) I am able to manage my anger every day.

0	1	2	3	4	5
not at all!					absolutely

3) I feel I have control over my reactions.

0	1	2	3	4	5
not at all!					absolutely

Want a FREE 30 minute coaching call with me?
When you're done reading – you'll learn how!

I know this stuff works for me!

I want to be sure it works for YOU!

So at the end of the book,

You'll see the section: A Quick Check-Out!

Here you'll answer the same 3 questions again!

We'll be able to tell if this

accomplishes what it is being written to do!

Give you more Anger Tools!

&

Get you managing ANGER daily!

See page 98 to see how you can

get a FREE 30 minute Consultation call with me!

Limited to the first 100 people

Part I

HOW to Get Started!

Where We Begin

Two birds are sitting on a wire.

One decides to fly away.

How many are left?

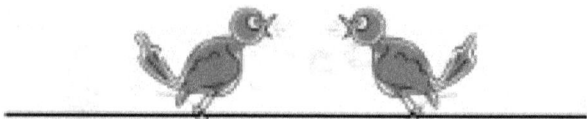

I like to start off my live workshops

with this little riddle.

It had such a tremendous impact on my life

the first time I heard it!

When they asked us to raise our hand

If we thought the answer was **one** -

My hand went up high & proud!

Wrong! The answer is two.

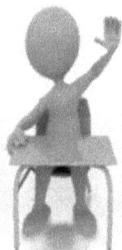

Oops!

DECIDING & DOING

are two different things!

Just because you decide to do something
DOESN'T mean that you DO it!

This was an ***Ah-Ha Moment*** for me -
There had been plenty of times

in my life when I **Decided**
&

I ***NEVER*** FOLLOWED
THRU!

What about you?

Do you have times when you've *DECIDED*
& NOT followed through like me?

(This little riddle *helped me change that!)*

This is my WordTool to get moving!

$$\mathbf{D}\text{irect}$$

$$\mathbf{O}\text{pportunity}$$

A quick note on WordTools!

I do not think these up rather **they come to me**,

usually inspired by someone or a situation....

I have learned to capture them when they show up!

I believe they can be tools to help us GROW!

The same rule applies to this

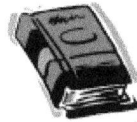

If you don't use what's in it,
it *won't work*.

KNOWING & DOING

are also two different things!

We either: DIRECT

opportunity

or

IT gets *directed for us!*

And chances are it WON'T take us in

a NEW direction with ***OUR ANGER!***

Is it worth the **COST***?*

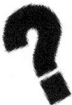

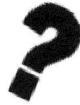

Here is what happens when we don't:

Denied

Opportunity

Not

'

Trying

Taken from "Words at Work"

There are also **many times** when we *don't get to control the cards we are dealt.in life.*

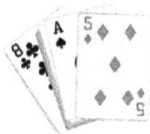

It's in these times of challenge when we need

to be *even BETTER able to manage ANGER!*

IT'S NOT

WHAT HAPPENS TO YOU,

BUT

HOW YOU REACT TO IT

THAT MATTERS

EPICTETUS

Or another way I had a patient put it:

IF YOU
ALWAYS DO

WHAT YOU'VE
ALWAYS DONE

YOU'LL
ALWAYS GET

WHAT YOU'VE
ALWAYS GOTTEN

BECAUSE IF
NOTHING CHANGES

*NOTHING
CHANGES!*

AUTHOR UNKNOWN

So before we move on to the next section,

I have a few rules I'd like to go over 1st.

They are critical to *your success*.

People don't usually have the chance to learn

these outside of *my* treatment programs.

So don't worry if you've never heard of them!

Carol's Rule #1

If we don't put words
to feelings –

***They come out as
behaviors...***

Carol's Rule #2

We have a right to
our feelings,

We ***don't*** have a right to
take them out on others!

Carol's Rule #3

DON'T

BLAME!

Here's what happens when we blame:

Become

Lost

Amongst

Many

Excuses!

Taken from "Words at Work"

It only tends to make things

WORSE!

When you put these 3 laws together,

they reinforce the

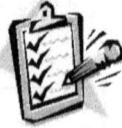

MOST important point when

it comes to dealing with anger:

WE are **responsible** for *our anger.*

No one *MAKES* us angry

No one *CAUSES* our anger

No one is the source

but **us!**

The fact you are reading this   right now

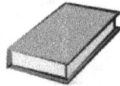

shows you are taking responsibility!

There are a couple quotes which ***helped me***

GET this important point that I'd like to share:

SMALL MINDED PEOPLE
BLAME OTHERS.

AVERAGE PEOPLE
BLAME THEMSELVES.

THE WISE SEE ALL BLAME

AS FOOLISHNESS.

EPICTETUS

ANY PERSON CAPABLE

OF *ANGERING YOU*

**BECOMES THE DRIVER OF
YOUR LIFE!**

CAROL RICKARD

I love the power of quotes!

You can sign up for a weekly equote at:

ThePowerofWordsEquote.com

Why ANGER Is *Not BAD*

Anger can be *a very powerful*

emotional stress response!

I would even argue it's **the most powerful!**

However, it *also gets a bad rap!*

There exists this myth that anger is

BAD

And you are a "bad" person if you get angry.

WRONG!

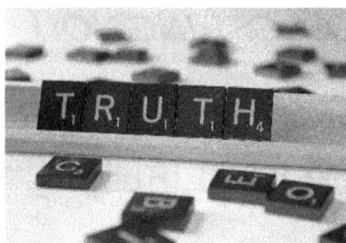

Anger is a natural emotion!

Emotions aren't **bad**.....

BEHAVIOR is!

Feelings & Behaviors are 2 *different* things & here's how they **FIT together!**

It came to me when I was doing a group on anger.

I asked members what they did when angry.

Joe replied:

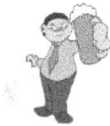

"I go to the bar & drink.
I can't help it."

What caught my attention was the

"I CAN'T HELP IT!"

You see, it might SEEM *like we can't help it* –

BUT we can!!!

And here's why"

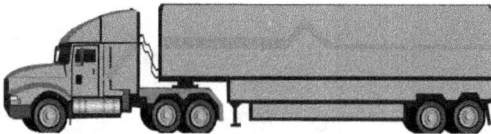

It seems to be one thing!

But is it?

29

When we take a closer look:

It's REALLY **2 parts!**

Just like our reactions have 2 parts!

FEELING   *BEHAVIOR:*

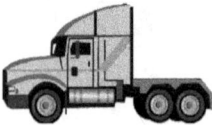   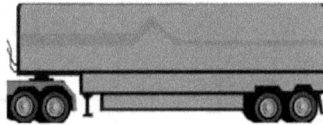

To Joe it feels like
his anger and his drinking are 1 thing!

The truth is they *are not!*

When we experience situations in life
that *"shake up"* FEELINGS in us......

It is up to us to CHOOSE

WHAT we will do with those FEELINGS!

We make the choice!

We decide which behavior we connect to!

**Joe's
ANGER**

ARGUE

DRINK

+ WAY

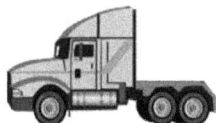

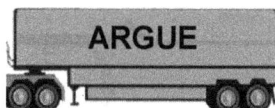

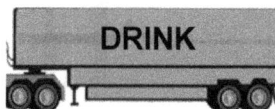

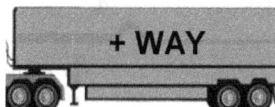

Which one will Joe CHOOSE!

(Which one will *you choose*!)

For the **1000's** I have shared this idea with –

it becomes an AH-HA
Moment!

WE are *responsible* for WHAT

WE DO with our feelings!

Here is the POWER of choice:

Controlling

How

Our

Intentions

Create

Experiences

YOU may need to make **NEW!** CHOICES

to deal with anger a better way

Don't set yourself up to fail!

The Secret to **SUCCESS:**

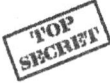

Choose a **new behavior**

you can **take action** on

Immediately!

Sadly,

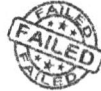

This is where I see most people......

get it WRONG!

They try to make *healthy changes* in their lives,

only to find themselves failing *miserably....*

Maybe this has happened to you in the past?

Again, it's one of those things I **only learned**

once I started working in treatment programs!

I love being able to share it with you!

Here's what I mean by this:

I asked Joe to pick one of the following
INSTEAD of "drinking" –

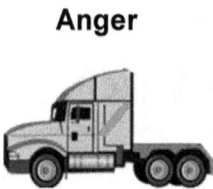
Support

Anger

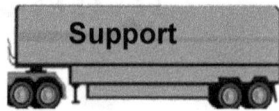

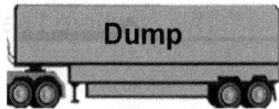
Dump

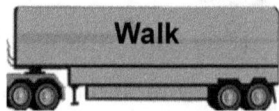
Walk

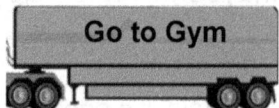
Go to Gym

These are all healthy LifeTOOLS!

His 1st pick was

"Go to Gym"

Then I asked:

"How long will it take to get to the gym?'

Joe replied, "It's a ½ hour from my house."

TOO LONG!!!!

How many places can Joe stop & drink on the way to the gym?!

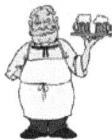

So I asked Joe to pick another!

His 2nd pick was

"Talk about it in my Support Group"

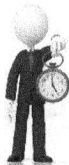

Still TOO LONG!!!!

WHY? It didn't meet until 3:00pm.

What happened if he got angry in the am?

So I hope you can see how Joe

was setting himself up to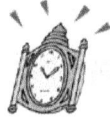

He was picking other ✚ ways

to *manage his anger!*

The **problem** is they weren't

things he could take action on

Immediately!!

The remaining two choices were both things he

COULD DO right away:

Anger

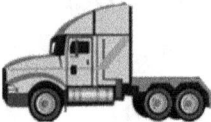

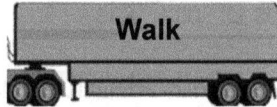

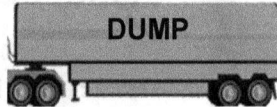

** I'll explain what *DUMPING* a little later!**

So it looks like one thing

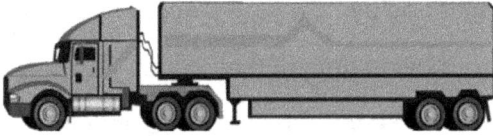

But it's important to remember –

IT'S NOT!!

FEELINGS & BEHAVIORS

Are 2 *Different*

things!!

This can be a **very powerful** concept to teach children.

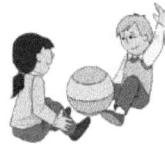

By helping them understand this early on –

We can then go on to teach them

healthier ways of coping with their feelings!

The Take Away's!

So, it's my hope by now you're able to see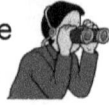
how to set yourself up for
Success from the very beginning!

TAKE AWAY
#1

We MUST take action -

DECIDING & *DOING*

Are 2 different things!

TAKE AWAY
#2

We get to CHOOSE -

FEELING 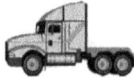   BEHAVIOR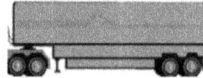

Are 2 different things!

TAKE AWAY
#3

We are RESPONSIBLE -

IT IS *OUR* FEELING.

It is our job to *MANAGE IT!*

Part II
WHAT It Looks Like

ALL Anger Is NOT the Same

In my **25** years of working with people,

I've identified **3 basic ways** ANGER

comes out!

I'm going to first introduce them to you, then

I'll go on to explain each one in more detail!

Up first is "The Boiler"`:

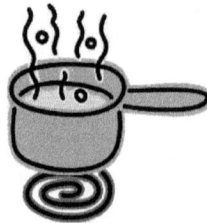

Next is "The Exploder":

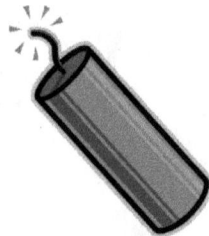

Last is "The Imploder":

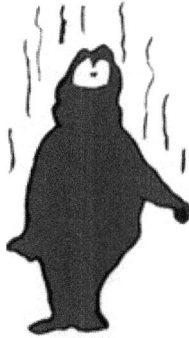

Just going by the pictures...

Is there one you think BEST describes you?

It's always interesting because I find when I'm

doing this in a workshop or a group,

people will often *immediately* identify which one

they think is them!

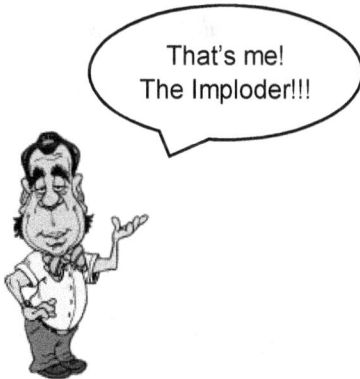

That's me!
The Imploder!!!

I call these **Anger STYLES**

So now I'll explain each one!

I want you to pay attention to which style you

think sounds **most** like what goes on with you.

KEY POINT:

Our focus is on

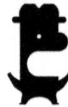

HOW your anger *COMES OUT*.

Often times,

People get hung up & they'll say:

"I don't really get angry".

I understand that! (More on this later!)

What I want you to think about is

WHEN you do -

Which style captures it best!

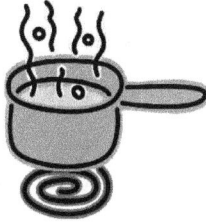

The Boiler

Leaves a small mess

No real *damage* to the situation

If you've ever had a pot *BOIL OVER* –

You know there is a **small mess** to clean up!

This is a key characteristic of

The Boiler

?   **?**

Are you the kind of person who

has anger come out at times and when it does,

it sort of gently *spills over?*

2nd - style

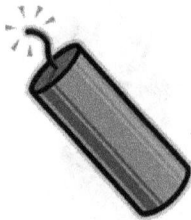

The Exploder

Leaves a medium to large mess

There is real damage to the situation -

especially relationships & environment.

If you've ever got to see on TV an *EXPLOSION* –

You know there's always **a mess** left behind!

This is a key characteristic of

The Exploder

? Are you the kind of person who **?**

has anger come out at times and when it does,

it has such power it **comes flying out?**

44

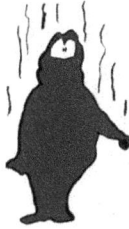

The Imploder

Leaves **YOU** as the "mess"!

There is ***damage to your health*** –

physical health & mental health

If you've ever seen a pipe BURST –

You know there's always **a mess** left behind!

This is a key characteristic of

The Exploder

?   **?**

Are you the kind of person who

holds all anger inside, where it never comes out

and it ***Makes you SICK?***

BEWARE!

Different situations may

trigger different responses!

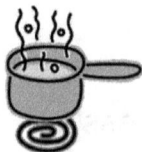

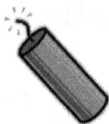

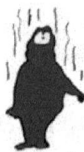

You could have **MORE** than 1 style!

Meet Sue!

She identified herself as **The Boiler!**

However, after talking about how

situations could trigger different styles –

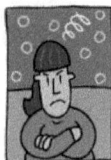

She quickly added:

"When I go to the motor vehicles division &

they are DISRESPECTFUL to me –

I get so angry they have

to **call the police**.*"*

46

Through our discussion....

Sue was able to realize that each time she has

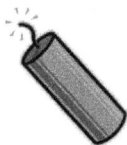

exploded

It's been when someone disrespected her.

We'll talk about BUTTONS a little later.

Just Sue having this information and *realizing the connection* meant she could

Change the outcomes!

After all,

YOU *DON'T KNOW*

WHAT *YOU DON'T KNOW*

UNTIL YOU LEARN

YOU DON'T KNOW IT!

CAROL L RICKARD

What About You?

Circle which Anger STYLE is your *primary* one:

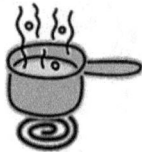

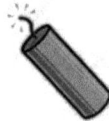

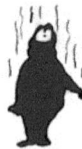

"Boiler"   **"Exploder"**   **"Imploder"**

Please take a moment to think about whether

there are *situations when this changes?*

If so, complete the following:

The Situation(s)	Your Anger STYLE
_____	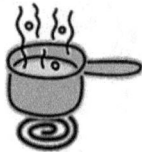 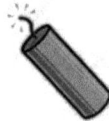 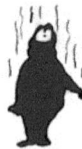
_____	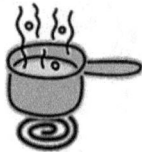 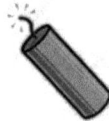 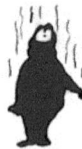
_____	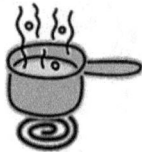 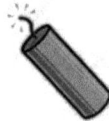 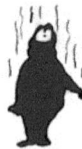

Many people are often surprised at what they see!

Many can actually be ALL 3

depending on situation!

Another Important Question ❓

So now that you know your **STYLE(S)** –

The *next* *IMPORTANT* **question** *to answer:*

How much time do you have?

If you're a

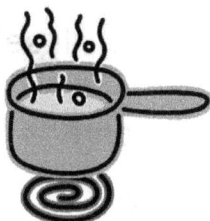

Check off which describes you:

Are you "*slow*" boiler?   _____

or

Are you "*quick*" boiler?   _____

Does the situation make a difference? Describe:

```



```

If you're an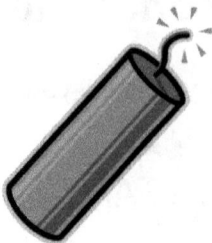

Check off which describes you:

Is your "fuse":

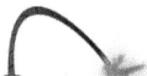 Long _____

or

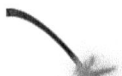 Medium _____

or

Short _____

Does the situation make a difference? Describe:

If you're an

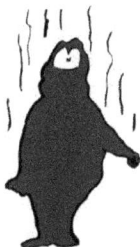

Check off which describes you:

How long can you "hold things in":

A little while _____

or

A *long* time _____

Does the situation make a difference? Describe:

> [blank box]

FYI! *It's not uncommon for IMPLODERS*

to have an occasional EXPLOSION...

Before we move on,

   please take a moment & write down below a

few things you've learned about anger so far!

Our brains hold on better to ideas

when they're written!

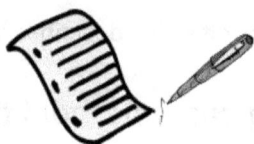

The Anger Umbrella

Good job getting to this point!

Anytime we stop and take a look at ourselves,

it can be ***challenging to do....***

That's why MOST people stay STUCK

&
don't continue to GROW!

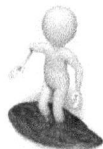

My hope is you've discovered some new things

about yourself when it comes to your anger.

I am pretty sure you'll discover some more things

in these next two sections!

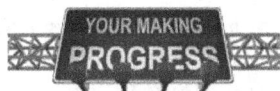

We are going to focus next on words,

or I should say

Anger Vocabulary

I'd like to share how I 1st came up with

"The Anger Umbrella"

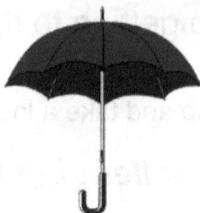

When I worked in Somerset hospital,

as part of my assessment I would ask people:

"What do you do when you get angry?"

I had this one little old lady who said to me:

"Oh, I don't get angry."

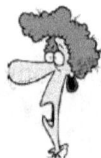

I said,

"Okay. What if your son says he is coming

*to visit and then he **never shows up** –*

how do you feel then?"

Her response:

"I feel upset."

That was an **Ah-ha moment** for me!

I realized for the 1st time:

People use *different words* to

identify their anger!

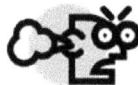

Each of us has our own

Anger Vocabulary!

So,

In order for us to **better manage** our anger –

we better know what to look out for!

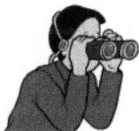

And we are now going to do that!

On the following pages,

I am going to help you identify yours!

Introducing the

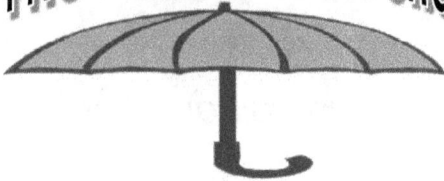

The Anger Umbrella

I've come to learn in my **25** years of working with

people there are **many** *different words* related

to anger that fit under *an umbrella of anger*!

IMPORTANT:

It's ***not*** what you DO…

It's the *word you use to describe* how you **FEEL**!

Remember, they are two different things!

Feeling   *Behavior*

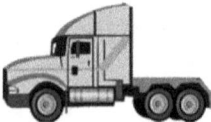   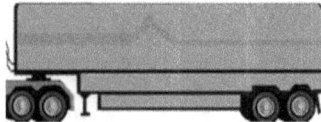

Directions:

Please take a few moments & write down

under the picture below as many words as you can

think of that **YOU *use* -** For example:

Do you get ***mad*** or ***angry***? Or do you get ***pissed off***

Do you get ***upset, frustrated,*** or ***irate?***

The Anger Umbrella

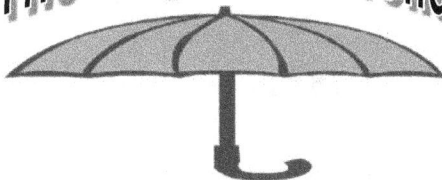

Remember: Only write words that describe the **feeling**!
NOT what you would DO

Good work! Now I want to help you see if there are any you might have forgotten.

1) Read through the list below.

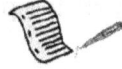

2) When you come to one that is a word you could see *yourself saying* – add it to your other ones!

Annoyed	Disrespected
Aggravated	Agitated
Jealous	Irate
Embarrassed	Ballistic
Overwhelmed	Let down
Upset	Hurt
Discouraged	Rage
Tense	Vindictive
Hateful	Argumentative
Pissed off	Inpatient
Mad	Perturbed
Stressed	Furious
Steamed	Disgusted
Disappointed	Confused
Sad	Powerless
Disgruntled	Livid
Defensive	Anxious
Betrayed	Depressed

What We've Done

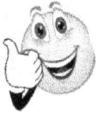

Congratulations!

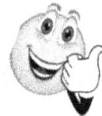

Here is the great work you've done so far:

1st You've identified your *primary*

Anger STYLE

2nd You've identified your

Anger VOCABULARY

Now, we want to take and build on this work!

The goal of this next step is for you to

REALLY get to know your anger!

3rd You'll identify your

Anger PATTERN

Figuring Out Your Pattern

There are basically two ways to approach
looking at & identifying your Anger PATTERN

#1- Focus on a specific situation where
your anger is getting the best of you.

#2- Focus on the general pattern your
anger tends to take on in your life.

NEXT:

Using your Anger VOCABULARY -
fill in the diagram that fits your style!

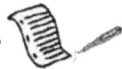

The Boiler – *"What's Your Boiling Point?"*

The Exploder – *"How Long Until You Explode?"*

The Imploder – *"What's Your Implosion Point?"*

60

Let's look at some examples!

Here is Steve's:

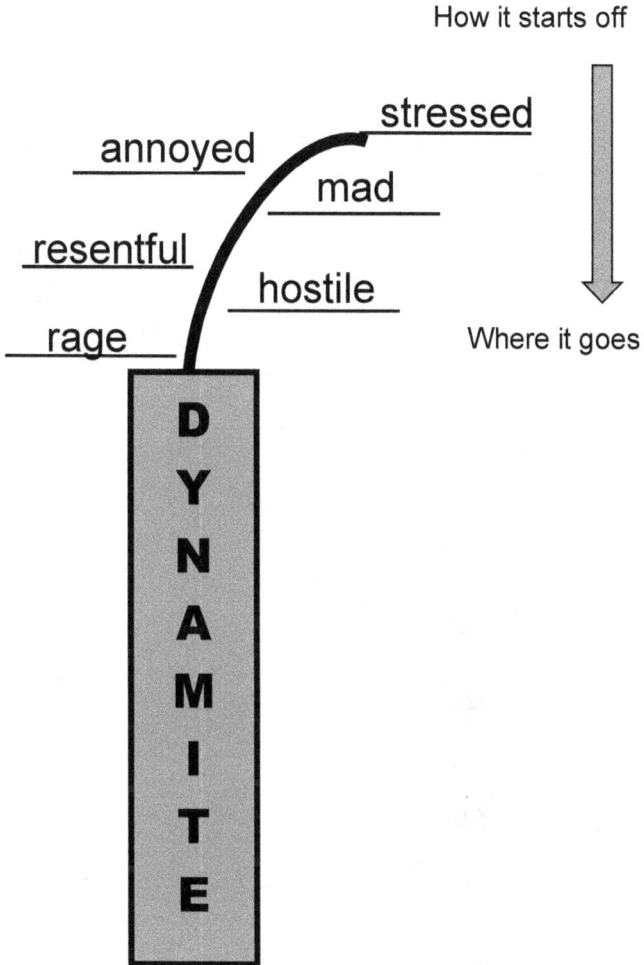

How it starts off

stressed

annoyed

mad

resentful

hostile

rage

Where it goes

DYNAMITE

A Long fuse

Here is Sue's pattern.

You'll see she has a **very short** fuse

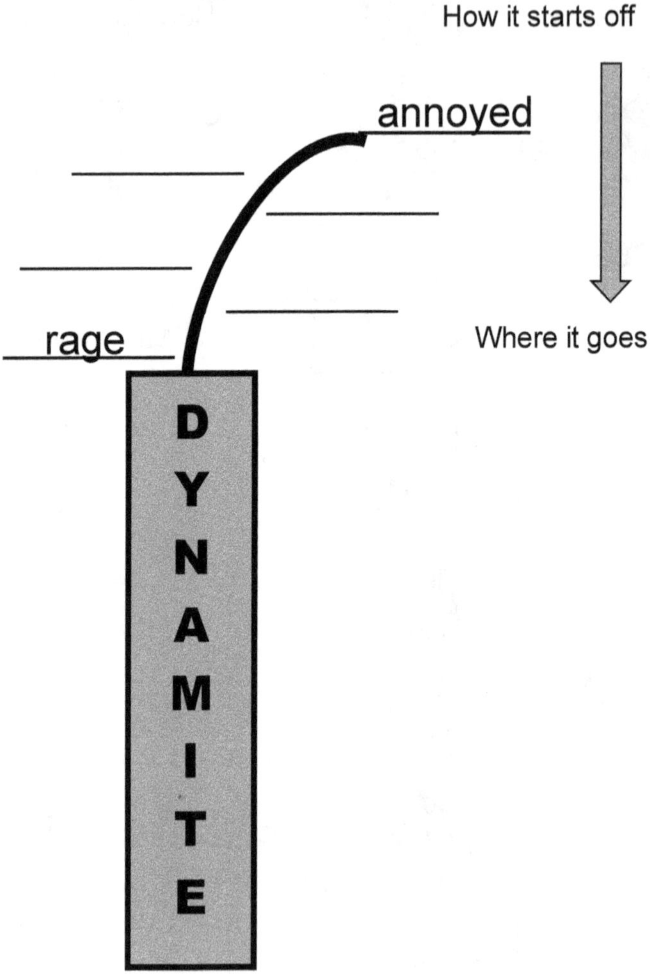

How it starts off

annoyed

_____

_____

_____

_____

rage

D
Y
N
A
M
I
T
E

Where it goes

A Short fuse

Boiler / Imploder Examples

The same thermometer works for both styles!

Here is Janet's:

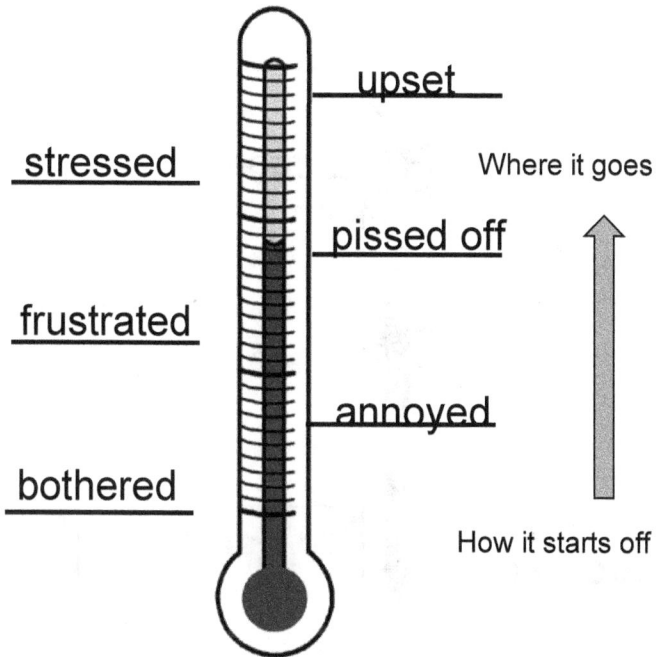

stressed

frustrated

bothered

upset

pissed off

annoyed

Where it goes

How it starts off

Slow

This is Dave's pattern.

You'll see he can be a **fast boil**:

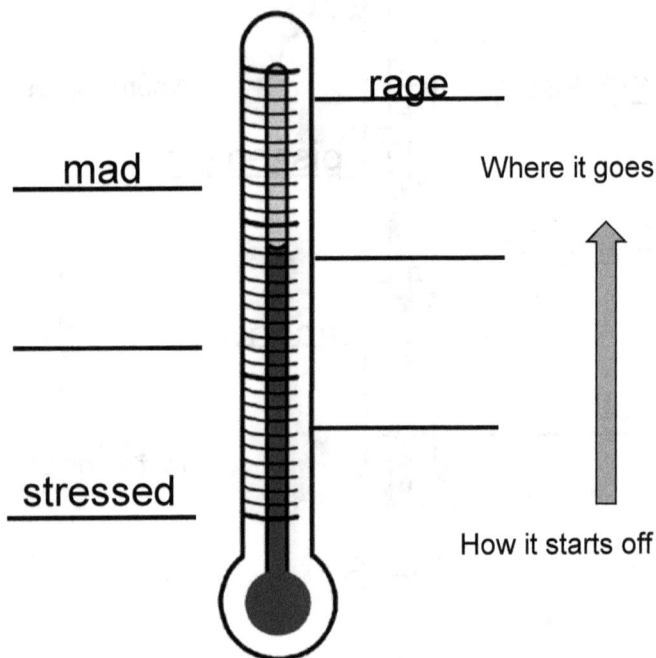

rage

mad

stressed

Where it goes

How it starts off

Fast

A few things I want you to *notice*:

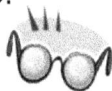

#1   Depending on "*how much time you have*",

you may not use *all* of the lines.

#2   There are no right or wrong answers!

This is you getting to see your anger.

#3   The *words don't all mean the same to us!*

You see stressed in two different places.

One place it is **low** & the other it is **high** –

This is why we can't assume when someone says

a feeling that we know what it means! **

So now it's your turn!

Using ONLY your vocabulary –

Fill in the action sheet that fits your

Anger STYLE

How Long Until You EXPLODE?

The situation: _____

There are 2 ways to approach this:

1) How does it START & then progress.

2) How does it END & move backwards.

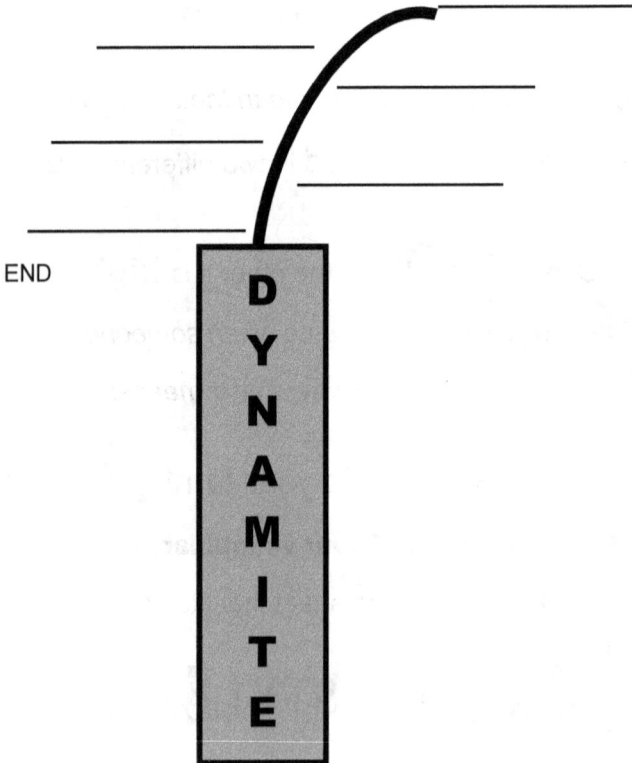

START

END

D
Y
N
A
M
I
T
E

What's Your
BOILING / IMPLOSION
Point?

The situation: _____

There are 2 ways to approach this:

1) How does it START & then progress.

2) How does it END & move backwards.

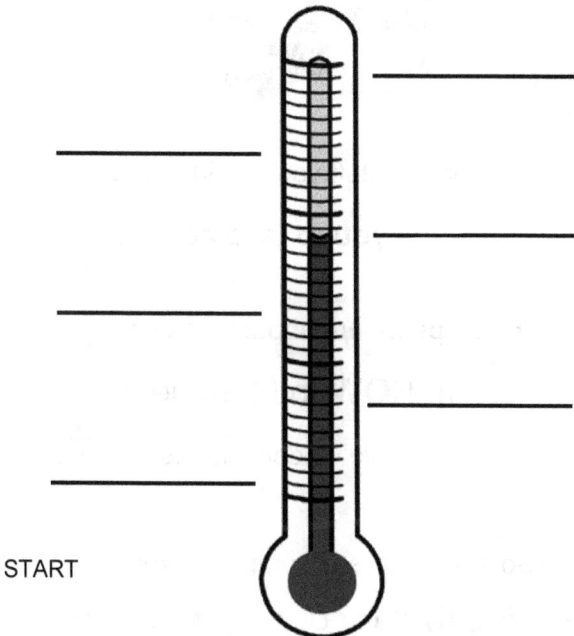

What Next?

CONGRATULATIONS!

If you've been completing the action sheets,

you are on *your way* to new success!

If you haven't –

I can promise - you are **not likely to see**

any changes happen in your life....

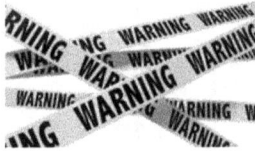

This is not the kind of stuff you can just read *about*!

It requires you to take action!

The steps we are about to take in

Part III: **HOW** to Manage It

Builds off of what we've done in this section!

(So, if you haven't completed your

anger vocabulary or **anger pattern** –

please go back now & do it!)

Part III

HOW to Manage It

The Secret!

When it comes to managing our anger

the secret is quite simple!

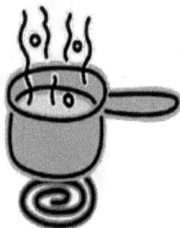

Catch it *BEFORE* it *boils over!*

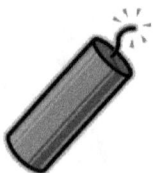

Catch it *BEFORE* it *explodes!*

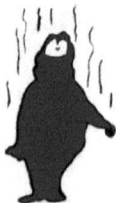

Catch it *BEFORE* it *implodes!*

I have created a no fail system

that when followed will lead you

to SUCCESS every time!

Carol's 2 Steps to Success!!

Yes! It really is that simple…

Just 2 steps is all it takes to begin to

MANAGE anger rather than IT

MANAGING you!

Where most people FAIL

Is that they *only do 1 step*.

Let's take a look at an example of this

on the next page:

71

Pete was already having a **difficult day** at work.

It started that morning when his

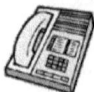 coworker called out.

Then his boss, not even realizing they were

shorthanded, gave Pete a job he wanted

done right away.

The stress of things started to get to Pete…

He could feel himself starting to get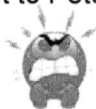

So to avoid things coming out & creating a BIG

mess, **he walked away** & finished in his office.

As he drove home,

he was *feeling pretty good* about his day.

He walked through his front door

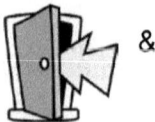 &

almost slipped on the toys left on the floor –

HE LOST IT…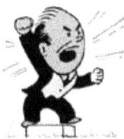

He started **yelling at the kids,**

who were actually playing

nicely at the table.

After he had *sent the kids to their rooms,*

he sat down & talked to his wife.

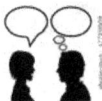

It was only then, in that moment, when he *realized*

He'd overreacted to the situation…

Yes, he was *upset* he almost fell.

Yes, he was *scared* he almost fell.

But most importantly -

he realized he was STILL *angry* from work.

He went to each of the kids & **apologized:**

"Daddy's sorry for yelling at you.

You didn't deserve that.

Daddy had a bad day at the office

and unfairly took it out on you two."

Has this EVER happened to you?

Stuff *spills out* on the wrong person?

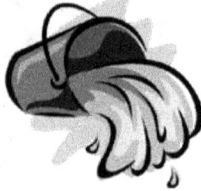

If Pete had DONE the 2nd step

He could have AVOIDED this mess at home!

So, let's move on to taking a look at:

Carol's 2 Steps to Success!!

Carol's 2 Steps to Success!!

Step 1

STOP the level from rising

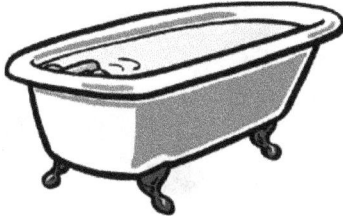

If we don't 1st **STOP** the level from rising

It will spill over!

How do we do this?

Do something *CALMING.*

The key here is it's something that is ***passive***.

(We'll look at some examples in a moment!)

Next.....

Step 2

RELEASE what's there!

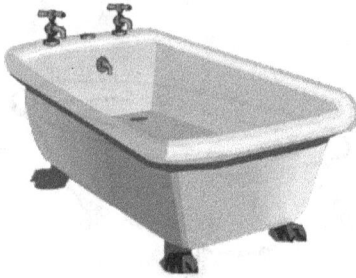

If we don't **then *RELEASE*** what's there

It will **spill over** when turned on again!

How do we do this?

Do something *ACTIVE.*

The key here is it's something that is ***active***.

(We'll look at some examples in a moment!)

76

As you can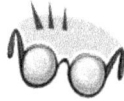

To have success requires we

DO *BOTH* STEPS!

PASSIVE: This refers to any activity that *does not* require any muscles be used.

ACTIVE: This refers to any activity that *DOES* require muscles be used!

If we go back & look at Pete's situation,

Can you see how by *walking away* –

He did STEP 1…

But by **NOT** doing STEP 2

He had no room to contain feeling *upset & scared*

So it *spilled over* on to the kids.

Ways to **STOP** the level from rising

Remove yourself

Go in to another area / place

Breathing

Concentrate on your breath

Do belly breathing,

Count to 10

Even better is counting each breath

Music

Listen to something that is very soothing

Meditation

Set a timer for a few minutes

Prayer

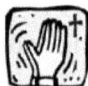

If this applies, it can be powerful!

Time out

Goes beyond just removing yourself

Focus attention elsewhere for set time

Guided imagery

Use your mind & imagination to go to relaxing place

Listen to a guided audio track

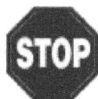

Thought stopping

Close your eyes for moment

Picture a giant stop sign in your mind!

+ Self-talk

Keep telling yourself + thoughts

Use one from our list on page 97

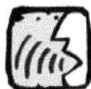

Serenity Prayer

Can I do anything about it now?

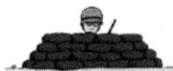

Mental Fox Hole

Imagine you're in a favorite place

Be there w/ all 5 senses

(see, hear, smell, feel, taste)

Reframing **

Ways of changing your thinking!

** Don't take it personal

Don't take on their crap

** It Is what It Is

Don't make it bigger with thoughts

Let Go

Listen to something that is very soothing

Hot shower/bath

Let yourself soak & enjoy

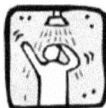

Aromatherapy

Use scents that are calming

Can be in a lotion or infuser!

Candles

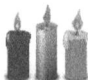

Can be just watching the flame

Can be enjoying the scent.

Self-Care

Make sure you are putting you 1st

Do something nice for yourself

Nature

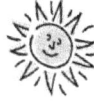

Look at it on your computer

Go look out a window / GO outside

Remember –

The key with all these is that they are all

Passive

Meaning they *DO NOT* require

any energy or muscle movement!

Step 1 – STOP levels from rising!

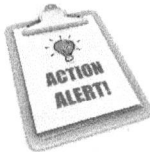

ACTION ALERT:

Go back through the list & **put a mark** next

to each one you are willing to try!

"The Quick 3" Stoppers!

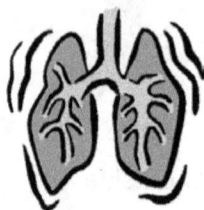

Breathe

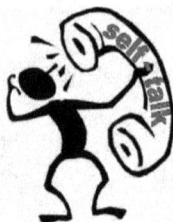

+ Self Talk

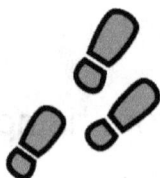

**Remove
yourself**

I call these the "emergency brakes"!

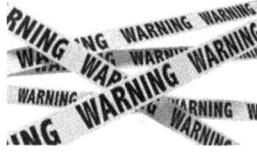

You CANNOT go on to Step 2

unless

You have **COMPLETED** Step 1

We must STOP the level from rising first!

Research has shown that if a person

HAS NOT 1st STOPPED the level from rising,

trying to "release" will only make them angrier.

This is why it's called

Carol's 2 Steps to Success!!

Step 1   **STOP**

Step 2   **RELEASE**

Ways to what's there!

Talk

Get together with someone you trust

Talk about your feelings – **not** *the situation*

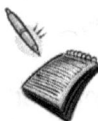

Write / Dumping

This is all about putting feelings on paper.

Can include writing a letter but NOT MAILING!

Punching Bag

Can be a heavy bag or a pillow.

There's even an adult inflatable one!

(If you had a Bozo the clown, you'd like this!)

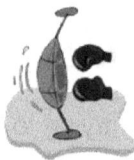

Clean

This has to be something that works for you!

Otherwise, it could make you angrier…

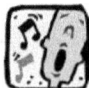

Sing / Play Air Instrument

Best way to turn music in to a 'release'!

Exercise

This can be at a gym or fitness center.

It's also doing other activity: i.e. sit up / push up

Pace

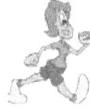

Walking up & down a hallway, stairwell or office

Scream in the car

Make sure the windows are up & let it ROAR!

Constructive Destruction

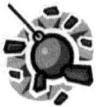

Destroy things on purpose:

Old dishes, furniture, etc.

Empty Chair Method

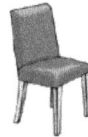

Taking to a chair as if a person was there.

Also good to do in the car as if there!

Cry

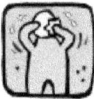

Let the tears flow....

Yoga

Take a class & try it out! You can do this anywhere.

Call Someone

Either fiend, family member, or help line

Texting does not count!

Tear up a phone book

Keep some old phone books on hand!

Laughter

This can be a great way of letting energy out!

Try a laughter yoga class

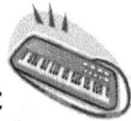

Play a musical instrument

This is an excellent way to discharge energy

Air Box

Don't have a heavy bag or punching bag?

This works too!

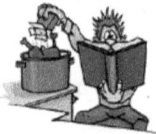

Cooking

Only if this works for you!

Gardening

This can indoor or outdoor! Be ACTIVE

Remember –

The key with all these is that they are all

ACTIVE

Meaning they *DO require*

energy or muscle movement!

Step 2 – RELEASE what's there!

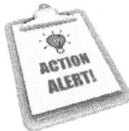 **ACTION ALERT:**

Go back through the list & **put a mark** next

to each one you are willing to try!

Are there any more you can think of?

If so, write them in down below:

"The Quick 3" Releases!

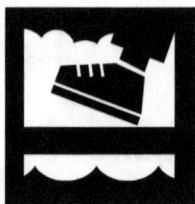

Walk

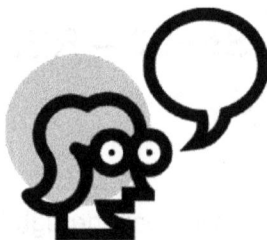

Talk

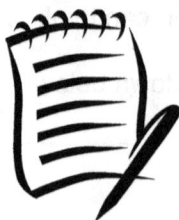

Write / Dump

A quick word on "dumping":

Dumping is when you write but

you **DON'T read** what you wrote!

Instead you destroy it!

There are a couple of ways you can *destroy it:*

Burn it

Shred it

Tear it up in to little pieces

Use toilet paper, sharpie & ***flush it***

Make a DUMP Box!

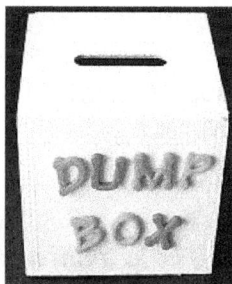

My story:

I once got so angry in a staff meeting,

it was all I could do to fight back the tears.

I felt betrayed, hurt, and disrespected.

As I drove home,

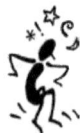

the more I thought about my boss,

the more pissed off I got!

When it came time to go to bed that night,

all my brain wanted to do was

"think" about my boss!

I was *finally able* to go to sleep AFTER

I wrote down my bosses name on a piece of paper

DUMPING IT

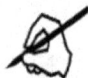

And fed in to a shredder!

The Take Away's!

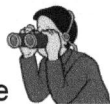

So, it's my hope by now you're able to see

how to MANAGE the anger & why it takes

2 Steps to Success!!

TAKE AWAY
#1

We must 1st STOP

the level from rising!

Passive

TAKE AWAY
#2

We must *then* RELEASE

what is there!

ACTIVE

TAKE AWAY
#3

We might need to do each step

more than once!

These steps only work when you *DO* them!

Dealing with Button Pushers

There are people in your life *who*:

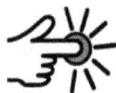

Know what buttons to push

Seem to **like** pushing your buttons

Will ***keep*** *trying to push your buttons!*

How do you STOP them?

YOU

DON'T!

You have **no more control** over them

than you do the **weather!**

You can save yourself a lot of work

by not even trying…

So what are you supposed to do?

Disconnect the wiring!

Let me share a true story -

When I was a young girl,

my brother & I went to the neighbor's house.

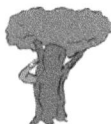

We'd ring the doorbell, RUN,

& hide behind a tree!

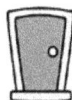

We'd watch as this older man would **open the door,**

look around and then go back inside.

After a few minutes, we'd do it again!

We kept doing it *UNTIL*

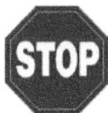

he STOP coming to the door....

The same principle applies when dealing with

Button Pushers

As long as they continue to get the reaction,

They will **keep** pushing!

The key is to

STOP giving them what they want:

Your
reaction!

Using your new

2 Steps to Success!!

you no longer have to REACT.

Instead,

You can disconnect the wiring!

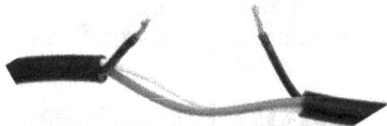

Earlier in the book, I shared Sue's story

about how she became "The Exploder"

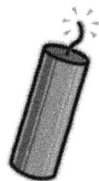

when her "disrespected" button got pushed.

Using the TOOLS you just learned –

Sue was able to *DISCONNECT* the old wiring

&

Respond in a whole new way!

In order to be able to disconnect the wiring

You must know what the buttons are!

On the next page,

I want you to identify a few of your buttons.

So, take a few moments and think about

who are your button pushers!

WHO PUSHES YOUR BUTTONS?

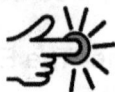

Who Does It?	Reaction - (Old Wiring)	New Wiring Response
_____	_____	_____
_____	_____	_____
_____	_____	_____
_____	_____	_____

(You can turn to page 99 if you need some examples!)

The Take Away!

We can't STOP button pushers.

Only our reaction to them

by using new tools!

+ Self-Talk Examples

Today I feel peace & calm.

I am free from past mistakes in my life.

I am free of old negative feelings.

I have all the time that I need.

My past no longer haunts me.

I am having a great day!

I am terrific just the way I am!

I no longer give my power to others.

I am getting better one step at a time.

I am learning to manage my emotions.

I deserve to be treated with love & respect.

I am doing the best I can for now.

Things could be worse!

I get there when I get there.

I can only try to change myself

A Quick Check- Out!

So I said this would be again at the end!
Circle the number below each statement that best
describes where you are RIGHT NOW!

1) I think people can be resistant or in denial that they need to change.

0	1	2	3	4	5

not at all!   absolutely

2) I think all a person needs to do is make up their mind to change & they can be successful.

0	1	2	3	4	5

not at all!   absolutely

3) I can get so busy helping others that I forget to take care of myself.

0	1	2	3	4	5

not at all!   absolutely

BONUS:
Send me an email with before & after scores!
I'll give you a 30-minute coaching call with me!!!

Carol@WellYOUniversity.com   Subject: ANGER
Limited number of slots available!

WHO PUSHES YOUR BUTTONS?

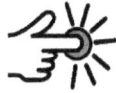

Examples:

Who Does It?	Reaction - (Old Wiring)	New Wiring Response
Husband	Argue	Talk
Wife	Curse	Walk Away
Aunt	Yell back	Laughter
Parent	Shutdown	Say No!
Boss	Migraines	Dump
Neighbors	Passive - aggressive	Assertive Communication
Drivers	Migraines	+ Self Talk
Passengers	Pain goes up	Sing

About the Author

Carol L Rickard, LCSW, TTS, of Hopewell, NJ is founder & CEO of WellYOUniversity, LLC, a global health education company dedicated *to empowering individuals with the tools and supports to achieve lifelong wellness & recovery.*

Also known as **America's Wellness Ambassador**, Carol is a dynamic & engaging speaker who brings to life practical / useful solutions. She is a weekly contributor for Esperanza Magazine; written 13 books on stress and wellness, had a guest appearance on Dr. Oz last year

She is also the creator & host of a 30-minute wellness show on Princeton TV - **The WELL YOU Show** which can be seen at:

www.TheWELLYOUShow.com

Get more of Carol at:

Twitter: ***@wellYOUlife***

"Like us" @ www.FaceBook.com/WellYOUniversity

Have Carol Speak at Your Next Event!

Get more information about how you can have Carol speak at your organization, event, or conference.

Go to: www.CarolLRickard.com

Or call: 888 Life Tools (543-3866)

Carol's Other Books

Help

Selfness

Stress Eating

Stretched Not Broken

The Caregiver's Toolbox

Transforming Illness to Wellness

Putting Your Weight Loss on Auto

The Benefits of Smoking

Moving Beyond Depression

LifeTools

Words At Work Vol. 1

Words at Work Vol. 2

Creating Compliance

Relapse Prevention

Please visit us at:

www.WellYOUniversity.com

Sign up for weekly motivational e-quote!

Check out our upcoming FREE webinars!

Learn more about our training programs.

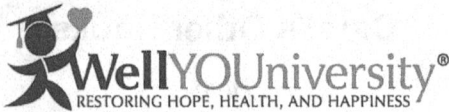

Email us your success story at:

Success@WellYOUniversity.com

We'd like to ask for your feedback

Please check out the next page
if this book has been HELPFUL for you!

We'd love to hear from you!

Feedback Card

Please take a moment & provide us some

feedback about the book you just read &

how you feel *it benefited YOU!*

_____

_____

Tear along here

_____

_____

Name: _____

Best Phone #: _____

Can we use your comments in our publicity materials?
Yes / No

If OK with you, what's the best time to call you:_____

Thank You!

Scan or take a picture & email:
Carol@WellYOUniversity.com

Snail mail: Carol Rickard
5 Zion Rd., Hopewell, NJ 08535

103